I0490929

HEALING FROM WITHIN

A Friendly Guide to Dealing with Depression and Finding Happiness

Written By:

Oladejo Anuoluwapo

Table of Contents

Chapter Four: Treatment Options

- Types of treatment for depression

- Medications for depression

- Therapy for depression

- Alternative and complementary treatments for depression

Chapter Five: Managing Depression Long-Term

- Strategies for managing depression in the long term

- Creating a relapse prevention plan

- Lifestyle changes that can support mental health

- Finding meaning and purpose in life

Chapter Six: Supporting Someone with Depression

- How to support a loved one with depression

- What to say and what not to say to someone with depression

- Self-care for caregivers of someone with depression

Conclusion

Introduction

Depression is a common mental health disorder that affects millions of people worldwide. It can impact all aspects of life, including relationships, work, and daily functioning. Dealing with depression can be a challenging and complex journey, but it is important to know that there is help available.

In this guide, we will explore strategies for dealing with depression. We will cover topics such as understanding depression, seeking help, coping strategies, treatment options, managing depression long-term, and supporting someone with depression.

First, we will delve into understanding depression, including the signs and symptoms, causes, and risk factors. It's important to recognize the warning signs of depression, such as persistent sadness or loss of interest in activities, and understand the underlying factors that may contribute to its development.

Next, we will explore the importance of seeking help for depression. This may include talking to a mental health professional, seeking support from loved ones, or utilizing self-help strategies. We will also discuss the potential barriers to seeking help and ways to overcome them.

Coping strategies are essential for managing depression. We will explore various self-help techniques that can be effective in managing symptoms, such as exercise, relaxation techniques, and social support. We will also discuss ways to reduce stress and improve overall well-being.

Treatment options for depression will also be covered, including medication, therapy, and alternative treatments. It's important to know that there are effective treatments available, and seeking professional help can significantly improve symptoms and quality of life.

Managing depression long-term requires ongoing effort and attention. We will discuss ways to maintain progress, such as self-monitoring, staying connected to support systems, and engaging in healthy behaviors.

Lastly, we will explore strategies for supporting someone with depression. Supporting a loved one with depression can be challenging, but it's essential to provide compassion, understanding, and encouragement.

In conclusion, this guide is intended to provide a comprehensive overview of depression and strategies for dealing with it. It's important to know that help is available, and recovery is possible. With the right tools and support, it is possible to manage depression and live a fulfilling life.

Chapter One: Understanding Depression

Depression is a common and serious mental health condition that can affect anyone, regardless of age, gender, or background. It is more than just feeling sad or down; depression can be a debilitating illness that impacts many aspects of a person's life, including their relationships, work, and physical health. In this chapter, we will explore what depression is, the different types of depression, the causes of depression, and the signs and symptoms to look out for.

What is Depression?

Depression is a mood disorder that affects a person's thoughts, feelings, and behavior. It is characterized by persistent feelings of sadness, hopelessness, and a lack of interest in things that were once enjoyable. Depression can range in severity from mild to severe, and it can last for weeks, months, or even years.

Types of Depression

There are several different types of depression, each with its own unique symptoms and causes. Some of the most common types of depression include:

1. Major Depressive Disorder: This is the most common type of depression, and it is characterized by persistent feelings of sadness, hopelessness, and a loss of interest in activities that were once enjoyable.

2. Persistent Depressive Disorder: This type of depression involves symptoms that are similar to major depressive disorder but are less severe and longer-lasting.

3. Seasonal Affective Disorder: This is a type of depression that occurs during the winter months when there is less sunlight. It is often characterized by feelings of sadness, fatigue, and social withdrawal.

4. Postpartum Depression: This type of depression can occur in women after giving birth and is characterized by feelings of sadness, anxiety, and exhaustion.

5. Bipolar Disorder: This is a type of depression that involves periods of extreme highs (mania) and extreme lows (depression).

Causes of Depression

Depression is a complex condition with multiple causes, and there is no one single factor that can cause depression. Some of the most common causes of depression include:

1. Genetics: Depression can run in families, indicating that there may be a genetic component to the condition.

2. Brain Chemistry: Imbalances in certain chemicals in the brain, such as serotonin and dopamine, can contribute to depression.

3. Life Events: Traumatic or stressful life events, such as the loss of a loved one or a job, can trigger depression.

4. Chronic Illness: People who have chronic health conditions, such as diabetes or heart disease, are more likely to develop depression.

5. Substance Abuse: Alcohol and drug abuse can contribute to depression, and people who have depression are more likely to turn to substance abuse as a way to cope with their symptoms.

Signs and Symptoms of Depression The symptoms of depression can vary from person to person, but some common signs to look out for include:

1. Persistent feelings of sadness, hopelessness, and helplessness

2. Loss of interest in activities that were once enjoyable

3. Fatigue and lack of energy

4. Changes in appetite and weight

5. Sleep disturbances, including insomnia or sleeping too much

6. Difficulty concentrating and making decisions

7. Feelings of worthlessness or guilt

8. Thoughts of suicide or self-harm

In conclusion, understanding depression is an important first step in dealing with the condition. By knowing the different types of depression, the causes of depression, and the signs and symptoms to look out for, individuals can better recognize the condition and seek the help they need. In the next chapter, we will explore how to seek help for depression and the different professionals who can assist with the condition.

Chapter Two: Seeking Help for Depression

If you're struggling with depression, it's important to know that you're not alone and that there is help available. Depression is a treatable condition, and seeking help is the first step towards feeling better. In this chapter, we will explore the different types of help available for depression, how to find the right mental health professional, and the different treatment options that can be effective in managing depression.

Types of Help Available There are several different types of help available for depression, and the type of help that's right for you will depend on your individual needs and circumstances. Some of the most common types of help available include:

1. Psychotherapy: This is a type of talk therapy that involves working with a mental health professional to explore and manage your feelings, behaviors, and thoughts. Psychotherapy can be effective in treating depression and is often used in conjunction with other treatments.

2. Medication: Antidepressant medication can be effective in managing depression, and there are several different types of antidepressants available. It's important to work closely with a healthcare professional

when taking antidepressants to manage potential side effects and ensure that the medication is effective.

3. Support Groups: Support groups can be an effective way to connect with others who are experiencing similar struggles with depression. Support groups can be found through mental health clinics, community centers, or online.

4. Self-Care: Self-care activities, such as exercise, meditation, and spending time with loved ones, can also be effective in managing depression. While self-care activities alone may not be enough to manage depression, they can be an important part of an overall treatment plan.

Finding the Right Mental Health Professional Finding the right mental health professional is an important step in managing depression. There are several different types of mental health professionals who can assist with depression, including:

1. Psychiatrists: Psychiatrists are medical doctors who specialize in treating mental health conditions, including depression. They can prescribe medication and provide therapy.

2. Psychologists: Psychologists are trained in diagnosing and treating mental health conditions and can provide therapy. They cannot prescribe medication.

3. Social Workers: Social workers can provide therapy and connect individuals with community resources to help manage depression.

4. Counselors: Counselors can provide therapy and support individuals in managing their depression.

Treatment Options for Depression There are several different treatment options available for depression, and the type of treatment that's right for you will depend on your individual needs and circumstances. Some of the most common treatment options include:

1. Cognitive Behavioral Therapy: This is a type of psychotherapy that focuses on changing negative thought patterns and behaviors that contribute to depression.

2. Interpersonal Therapy: This is a type of psychotherapy that focuses on improving communication and relationships to manage depression.

3. Medication: Antidepressant medication can be effective in managing depression, and there are several different types of antidepressants available.

4. Electroconvulsive Therapy (ECT): ECT is a medical procedure that involves the use of electrical currents to treat depression. It is often used in cases where other treatments have not been effective.

In conclusion, seeking help for depression is an important step in managing the condition. By understanding the different types of help available, finding the right mental health professional, and exploring the different treatment options, individuals can take control of their depression and work towards feeling better. In the next chapter, we will explore self-care strategies that can be effective in managing depression.

Chapter Three: Coping Strategies for Depression

While seeking professional help and treatment is essential for managing depression, there are also many coping strategies that individuals can use to manage their symptoms and improve their overall well-being. In this chapter, we will explore a range of coping strategies that can be effective in managing depression.

1. Exercise: Regular exercise has been shown to be an effective way to manage depression. Exercise releases endorphins, which are natural chemicals in the brain that improve mood and reduce feelings of pain.

2. Mindfulness Meditation: Mindfulness meditation involves focusing on the present moment and accepting it without judgment. This can be an effective way to reduce stress and manage symptoms of depression.

3. Journaling: Writing down your thoughts and feelings can be a helpful way to manage depression. Journaling can help you identify negative thought patterns and find ways to challenge them.

4. Creative Expression: Engaging in creative activities such as painting, drawing, or writing can be an effective way to manage depression. Creative

expression allows individuals to channel their emotions into a productive and positive outlet.

5. Self-Care: Taking care of yourself is an essential part of managing depression. This includes getting enough sleep, eating a healthy diet, and taking time for activities that you enjoy.

6. Social Support: Having a support system of friends and family members can be an effective way to manage depression. Talking to someone you trust about your feelings can help you feel less alone and provide a sense of support.

7. Positive Self-Talk: Depression often involves negative self-talk and criticism. Learning to recognize negative self-talk and replace it with positive self-talk can be an effective way to manage depression.

8. Relaxation Techniques: Relaxation techniques such as deep breathing, progressive muscle relaxation, and visualization can be effective in managing depression by reducing stress and promoting feelings of calm.

9. Time Management: Managing your time effectively can help reduce feelings of overwhelm and stress, which can contribute to depression.

10. Gratitude Practice: Practicing gratitude by focusing on the positive aspects of your life can be an effective way to manage depression. This can be as simple as writing down three things you're grateful for each day.

It's important to remember that everyone's experience with depression is unique, and what works for one person may not work for another. It may take time to find the coping strategies that work best for you, but it's important to continue to explore and try different strategies until you find what works for you.

In conclusion, coping strategies can be an effective way to manage symptoms of depression and improve overall well-being. By engaging in self-care, social support, positive self-talk, relaxation techniques, and other coping strategies, individuals can take control of their depression and work towards feeling better. In the next chapter, we will explore how to support a loved one who is struggling with depression.

Chapter Four: Treatment Options for Depression

While coping strategies can be effective in managing symptoms of depression, some individuals may require additional treatment options to fully manage their depression. In this chapter, we will explore a range of treatment options available for individuals struggling with depression.

1. Therapy: Therapy is a common and effective treatment option for depression. Cognitive-behavioral therapy (CBT) and interpersonal therapy (IPT) are two types of therapy that have been shown to be effective in treating depression.

CBT focuses on changing negative thought patterns and behaviors that contribute to depression. Through CBT, individuals can learn to identify negative thought patterns and replace them with more positive and realistic ones.

IPT focuses on improving relationships and communication skills to help individuals manage depression. By improving interpersonal relationships, individuals can learn to better manage symptoms of depression.

2. Medication: Antidepressant medication is another treatment option for depression. There are several types of antidepressants available, and it may

take some trial and error to find the medication that works best for an individual.

It's important to note that medication is not a cure for depression and should always be used in conjunction with therapy and other coping strategies.

3. Electroconvulsive Therapy (ECT): ECT is a treatment option for severe cases of depression that do not respond to other treatments. During ECT, a small electrical current is applied to the brain while the individual is under anesthesia.

   ECT has been shown to be effective in treating severe depression, but it is usually only recommended when other treatments have not been successful.

4. Transcranial Magnetic Stimulation (TMS): TMS is a non-invasive treatment option that uses magnetic fields to stimulate nerve cells in the brain. TMS has been shown to be effective in treating depression, particularly in individuals who have not responded to medication.

5. Alternative Therapies: Alternative therapies such as acupuncture, yoga, and meditation can also be effective in managing depression. While the

effectiveness of these treatments has not been fully established through research, many individuals find them helpful in managing their depression.

It's important to work with a mental health professional to determine the best treatment options for managing depression. Treatment may involve a combination of therapy, medication, and other treatments based on an individual's unique needs.

In conclusion, there are several treatment options available for managing depression. Therapy, medication, ECT, TMS, and alternative therapies can all be effective in managing symptoms of depression. It's important to work with a mental health professional to determine the best treatment options for your unique needs.

Chapter Five: Managing Depression Long-Term

Managing depression can be a lifelong process. Even with effective treatment, individuals may experience periods of relapse or difficulty managing symptoms. In this chapter, we will explore strategies for managing depression long-term.

1. Consistent Treatment: Consistent treatment is important for managing depression long-term. This may include ongoing therapy, medication management, or other treatments recommended by a mental health professional.

It's important to keep up with treatment, even during periods where symptoms are not present. Skipping appointments or discontinuing medication can increase the likelihood of relapse.

2. Lifestyle Changes: Lifestyle changes can be helpful in managing depression long-term. This may include regular exercise, healthy eating habits, and getting enough sleep.

Exercise has been shown to be effective in managing depression. Even low-intensity exercise, such as walking, can have a positive impact on mood.

Healthy eating habits can also be helpful in managing depression. Consuming a balanced diet rich in fruits, vegetables, and whole grains can provide important nutrients that support overall health.

Getting enough sleep is also important for managing depression. Adequate sleep can help regulate mood and improve overall health.

3. Self-Care: Self-care is an important aspect of managing depression long-term. This may include engaging in activities that bring joy or relaxation, such as reading, taking a bath, or spending time in nature.

It's important to prioritize self-care and make time for activities that promote well-being. Self-care can help reduce stress and improve overall mood.

4. Support System: A support system can be instrumental in managing depression long-term. This may include family, friends, or support groups.

It's important to reach out to others and seek support when needed. Support can help individuals feel less isolated and provide a sense of connection.

5. Mindfulness Practices: Mindfulness practices, such as meditation or deep breathing, can be helpful in managing depression long-term. Mindfulness can help individuals stay present in the moment and reduce feelings of anxiety or stress.

Practicing mindfulness regularly can help individuals manage symptoms of depression and improve overall well-being.

In conclusion, managing depression long-term requires ongoing effort and commitment. Consistent treatment, lifestyle changes, self-care, a support system, and mindfulness practices can all be helpful in managing depression long-term. It's important to work with a mental health professional and implement strategies that work best for your unique needs.

Chapter Six: Supporting Someone with Depression

Supporting someone with depression can be challenging. It can be difficult to know what to say or how to help. In this chapter, we will explore strategies for supporting someone with depression.

1. Educate Yourself: Educating yourself about depression can help you better understand what your loved one is experiencing. It's important to learn about the symptoms of depression, how it can impact daily life, and treatment options.

2. Listen: It's important to listen to your loved one without judgment. Encourage them to talk about their feelings and concerns. Let them know that you're there to support them.

3. Be Supportive: Let your loved one know that you're there for them. Offer to help with everyday tasks, such as cooking or cleaning. Make time for activities that you can do together, such as going for a walk or watching a movie.

4. Encourage Treatment: Encourage your loved one to seek treatment for their depression. Offer to help them find a mental health professional or accompany them to appointments.

5. Be Patient: Recovery from depression can take time. It's important to be patient and understanding. Avoid placing pressure on your loved one to "get better" quickly.

6. Take Care of Yourself: Supporting someone with depression can be emotionally draining. It's important to take care of yourself as well. Make time for activities that you enjoy and seek support from friends and family.

7. Avoid Blaming or Shaming: Avoid blaming or shaming your loved one for their depression. Depression is a medical condition that requires treatment, not a personal failing.

8. Encourage Self-Care: Encourage your loved one to engage in self-care activities, such as exercise or meditation. Help them prioritize activities that promote well-being.

9. Seek Support: Supporting someone with depression can be challenging. It's important to seek support from others, such as a therapist or support group.

In conclusion, supporting someone with depression requires patience, understanding, and compassion. Educating yourself about depression, listening, being supportive, encouraging treatment, and taking care of yourself are all important strategies for supporting someone with depression. Remember to seek support for yourself and avoid blaming or shaming your loved one for their depression.

General Conclusion

In conclusion, dealing with depression can be a challenging and complex journey, but there are many strategies and resources available to help individuals manage their symptoms and improve their overall well-being.

Throughout this guide, we have explored several key topics related to depression, including understanding depression, seeking help, coping strategies, treatment options, managing depression long-term, and supporting someone with depression.

We have learned that depression is a medical condition that requires treatment, and seeking professional help from a mental health professional is essential. There are also many self-help strategies that can be effective in managing depression, including exercise, self-care, and stress reduction techniques.

It is important to recognize that recovery from depression can take time, and there may be setbacks along the way. However, with the right treatment and support, it is possible to manage depression and improve quality of life.

Remember, if you are struggling with depression, there is no shame in seeking help. You are not alone, and there are many resources available to support you on your journey towards wellness. Whether it's seeking professional help, talking to a trusted friend or family member, or engaging in self-care activities, know that there is hope for a brighter future.

With the right tools and support, it is possible to manage depression and live a fulfilling life. Always remember to prioritize your mental health, seek help when needed, and be kind to yourself throughout the process.

Thanks for Reading!